FATTY LIVER DIET

40+ Soup, Pizza, and Side Dishes recipes designed for Fatty Liver diet

TABLE OF CONTENTS

utter responsibility of the recipient reader. Under no circumstances will any legal responsibility or blame be held against the publisher for any reparation, damages, or monetary loss due to the information herein, either directly or indirectly.

Respective authors own all copyrights not held by the publisher.

The information herein is offered for informational purposes solely, and is universal as so. The presentation of the information is without contract or any type of guarantee assurance.

The trademarks that are used are without any consent, and the publication of the trademark is without permission or backing by the trademark owner. All trademarks and brands within this book are for clarifying purposes only and are the owned by the owners themselves, not affiliated with this document.

Introduction

Fatty Liver recipes for personal enjoyment but also for family enjoyment. You will love them for sure for how easy it is to prepare them.

ZUCCHINI SOUP

Serves: **4**

Prep Time: **10**   Minutes

Cook Time: **20**   Minutes

Total Time: **30**   Minutes

INGREDIENTS

- 1 tablespoon olive oil
- 1 lb. zucchini
- ¼ red onion
- ½ cup all-purpose flour
- ¼ tsp salt
- ¼ tsp pepper
- 1 can vegetable broth
- 1 cup heavy cream

DIRECTIONS

1. In a saucepan heat olive oil and sauté zucchini until tender

2. Add remaining ingredients to the saucepan and bring to a boil

3. When all the vegetables are tender transfer to a blender and blend until smooth

4. Pour soup into bowls, garnish with parsley and serve

Serves: **4**

Prep Time: **10**   Minutes

Cook Time: **20**   Minutes

Total Time: **30**   Minutes

INGREDIENTS

- **1 tablespoon olive oil**
- **1 lb. broccoli**
- **¼ red onion**
- **½ cup all-purpose flour**
- **¼ tsp salt**
- **¼ tsp pepper**
- **1 can vegetable broth**
- **1 cup heavy cream**

DIRECTIONS

1. In a saucepan heat olive oil and sauté broccoli until tender
2. Add remaining ingredients to the saucepan and bring to a boil
3. When all the vegetables are tender transfer to a blender and blend until smooth
4. Pour soup into bowls, garnish with parsley and serve

Serves: **4**
Prep Time: **10** Minutes
Cook Time: **20** Minutes
Total Time: **30** Minutes

INGREDIENTS

- 1 tablespoon olive oil
- 1 lb. tomato
- ¼ red onion
- ½ cup all-purpose flour
- ¼ tsp salt
- ¼ tsp pepper
- 1 can vegetable broth
- 1 cup heavy cream

DIRECTIONS

1. In a saucepan heat olive oil and sauté tomatoes until tender
2. Add remaining ingredients to the saucepan and bring to a boil
3. When all the vegetables are tender transfer to a blender and blend until smooth
4. Pour soup into bowls, garnish with parsley and serve

Serves: **4**
Prep Time: **10** Minutes

Cook Time: **20** Minutes

Total Time: **30** Minutes

INGREDIENTS

- 1 tablespoon olive oil
- ½ lb. onion
- ¼ red onion
- ½ cup all-purpose flour
- ¼ tsp salt
- 1 lb. carrot
- ¼ tsp pepper
- 1 can vegetable broth
- 1 cup heavy cream

DIRECTIONS

1. In a saucepan heat olive oil and sauté onion until tender
2. Add remaining ingredients to the saucepan and bring to a boil
3. When all the vegetables are tender transfer to a blender and blend until smooth
4. Pour soup into bowls, garnish with parsley and serve

Serves: **4**

Prep Time: **10**   Minutes

Cook Time: **20**   Minutes

Total Time: **30**   Minutes

INGREDIENTS

- 1 tablespoon olive oil
- 1 lb. carrot
- ¼ red onion
- ½ cup all-purpose flour
- ¼ tsp salt
- ¼ tsp pepper
- 1 can vegetable broth
- 1 cup heavy cream

DIRECTIONS

1. In a saucepan heat olive oil and sauté carrots until tender

2. Add remaining ingredients to the saucepan and bring to a boil

3. When all the vegetables are tender transfer to a blender and blend until smooth

4. Pour soup into bowls, garnish with parsley and serve

Serves: **4**
Prep Time: **10**   Minutes
Cook Time: **20**   Minutes
Total Time: **30**   Minutes

INGREDIENTS

- 1 tablespoon olive oil
- 1 lb. cucumber
- ¼ red onion
- ½ cup all-purpose flour
- ¼ tsp salt
- ¼ tsp pepper
- 1 can vegetable broth
- 1 cup heavy cream

DIRECTIONS

1. In a saucepan heat olive oil and sauté cucumber until tender
2. Add remaining ingredients to the saucepan and bring to a boil
3. When all the vegetables are tender transfer to a blender and blend until smooth
4. Pour soup into bowls, garnish with parsley and serve

Serves: *4*
Prep Time: *10* Minutes

Cook Time: *20* Minutes

Total Time: *30* Minutes

INGREDIENTS

- 1 tablespoon olive oil
- 1 lb. shallot
- ¼ red onion
- ½ cup all-purpose flour
- ¼ tsp salt
- ¼ tsp pepper
- 1 can vegetable broth
- 1 cup heavy cream

DIRECTIONS

1. In a saucepan heat olive oil and sauté shallot until tender

2. Add remaining ingredients to the saucepan and bring to a boil

3. When all the vegetables are tender transfer to a blender and blend until smooth

4. Pour soup into bowls, garnish with parsley and serve

Serves: *4*
Prep Time: *10*   Minutes

Cook Time: *20*   Minutes

Total Time: *30*   Minutes

INGREDIENTS

- 1 tablespoon olive oil
- 1 lb. corn
- ¼ red onion
- ½ cup all-purpose flour
- ¼ tsp salt
- ¼ tsp pepper
- 1 can vegetable broth
- 1 cup heavy cream

DIRECTIONS

1. In a saucepan heat olive oil and sauté corn until tender

2. Add remaining ingredients to the saucepan and bring to a boil

3. When all the vegetables are tender transfer to a blender and blend until smooth

4. Pour soup into bowls, garnish with parsley and serve

Serves: *4*
Prep Time: *10* Minutes
Cook Time: *20* Minutes
Total Time: *30* Minutes

INGREDIENTS

- 1 tablespoon olive oil
- 2 lb. red bell pepper
- ¼ red onion
- ½ cup all-purpose flour
- ¼ tsp salt
- ¼ tsp pepper
- 1 can vegetable broth
- 1 cup heavy cream

DIRECTIONS

1. In a saucepan heat olive oil and sauté red bell pepper until tender

2. Add remaining ingredients to the saucepan and bring to a boil

3. When all the vegetables are tender transfer to a blender and blend until smooth

4. Pour soup into bowls, garnish with parsley and serve

GREEN PESTO PASTA

Serves: *2*
Prep Time: *5*   Minutes
Cook Time: *15*   Minutes
Total Time: *20*   Minutes

INGREDIENTS

- 4 oz. spaghetti
- 2 cups basil leaves
- 2 garlic cloves
- ¼ cup olive oil
- 2 tablespoons parmesan cheese
- ½ tsp black pepper

DIRECTIONS

1. **Bring water to a boil and add pasta**

2. In a blend add parmesan cheese, basil leaves, garlic and blend

3. Add olive oil, pepper and blend again

4. Pour pesto onto pasta and serve when ready

Serves: **2**
Prep Time: **5**   Minutes
Cook Time: **15** Minutes
Total Time: **20** Minutes

INGREDIENTS

- 10 oz. spaghetti
- 2 eggs
- ½ cup parmesan cheese
- 1 tsp black pepper
- Olive oil
- 1 tsp parsley
- 2 cloves garlic

DIRECTIONS

1. In a pot boil spaghetti (or any other type of pasta), drain and set aside

2. In a bowl whish eggs with parmesan cheese
3. In a skillet heat olive oil, add garlic and cook for 1-2 minutes
4. Pour egg mixture and mix well
5. Add pasta and stir well
6. When ready garnish with parsley and serve

BEEF SPAGHETTI

Serves: **2**
Prep Time: **5**   Minutes

Cook Time: **15** Minutes

Total Time: **20** Minutes

INGREDIENTS

- **10 oz. spaghetti**
- **2 eggs**
- **1 lb. beef**
- **½ cup parmesan cheese**
- **1 tsp black pepper**
- **Olive oil**
- **1 tsp parsley**
- **2 cloves garlic**

DIRECTIONS

1. In a pot boil spaghetti (or any other type of pasta), drain and set aside
2. In a bowl whish eggs with parmesan cheese
3. In a skillet heat olive oil, add garlic and cook for 1-2 minutes
4. Pour egg mixture and mix well
5. Add pasta, cooked beef and stir well
6. When ready garnish with parsley and serve

SALMON PASTA

Serves: **2**
Prep Time: **5** Minutes
Cook Time: **15** Minutes
Total Time: **20** Minutes

INGREDIENTS

- 10 oz. spaghetti
- 2 eggs
- 1 lb. salmon
- ½ cup parmesan cheese
- 1 tsp black pepper
- Olive oil
- 1 tsp parsley
- 2 cloves garlic

DIRECTIONS

1. In a pot boil spaghetti (or any other type of pasta), drain and set aside
2. In a bowl whish eggs with parmesan cheese
3. In a skillet heat olive oil, add garlic and cook for 1-2 minutes
4. Pour egg mixture and mix well
5. Add pasta, salmon and stir well
6. When ready garnish with parsley and serve

CHICKEN SPAGHETTI

Serves: **2**

Prep Time: **5**   Minutes

Cook Time: **15**   Minutes

Total Time: **20**   Minutes

INGREDIENTS

- 10 oz. spaghetti
- 2 eggs
- 1 lb. cooked chicken breast
- ½ cup parmesan cheese
- 1 tsp black pepper
- Olive oil
- 1 tsp parsley
- 2 cloves garlic

DIRECTIONS

1. In a pot boil spaghetti (or any other type of pasta), drain and set aside
2. In a bowl whish eggs with parmesan cheese
3. In a skillet heat olive oil, add garlic and cook for 1-2 minutes
4. Pour egg mixture and mix well
5. Add pasta, cooked chicken breast and stir well
6. When ready garnish with parsley and serve

Serves: **2**
Prep Time: **5**   Minutes

Cook Time: **15** Minutes

Total Time: **20** Minutes

INGREDIENTS

- ½ cup celery
- 1 packet Knox Gelatin
- 1 cup cranberry juice
- 1 can berry cranberry sauce
- 1 cup sour cream

DIRECTIONS

1. **In a bowl combine all ingredients together and mix well**
2. **Add dressing and serve**

COBB SALAD

Serves: **2**

Prep Time: **5** Minutes

Cook Time: **15** Minutes

Total Time: **20** Minutes

INGREDIENTS

- 1 tablespoon mustard
- ¼ cup olive oil
- 1 head romaine lettuce
- 2 hard-boiled eggs
- 8 oz. bacon
- 1 avocado
- 6 oz. blue cheese
- 4 oz. tomatoes

DIRECTIONS

1. In a bowl combine all ingredients together
    and mix well
2. Add dressing and serve

Serves: 2
Prep Time: 5   Minutes
Cook Time: 15   Minutes
Total Time: 20   Minutes

INGREDIENTS

- 1 head cauliflower
- 4 slices bacon
- ¼ cup sour cream
- 1 tablespoon lemon juice
- ¼ tsp garlic powder
- 1 cup cheddar cheese
- 1 tablespoon chopped chives

DIRECTIONS

1. In a bowl combine all ingredients together and mix well

2. Add dressing and serve

Serves: 2
Prep Time: 5   Minutes
Cook Time: 15   Minutes
Total Time: 20   Minutes

INGREDIENTS

- 1 cup buffalo sauce
- 1 tablespoon honey
- 1 tsp lime
- 1 tsp salt
- 1 tsp onion powder
- 1 tablespoon olive oil
- 1 cup salad dressing

DIRECTIONS

1. In a bowl combine all ingredients together and mix well

2. Add dressing and serve

Serves: 2
Prep Time: 5   Minutes
Cook Time: 15   Minutes
Total Time: 20   Minutes

INGREDIENTS

- 1 cup farro
- 1 bay leaf
- 1 shallot
- ¼ cup olive oil
- 1 tablespoon apple cider vinegar
- 1 tsp honey
- 1 cup arugula
- 1 apple
- ¼ cup basil
- ¼ cup parsley

DIRECTIONS

1. In a bowl combine all ingredients together and mix well
2. Add dressing and serve

CARROT SALAD

Serves: **2**
Prep Time: **5** Minutes
Cook Time: **15** Minutes
Total Time: **20** Minutes

INGREDIENTS

- 1 lb. carrots
- 1 cup raisins
- ½ cup peanuts
- ½ cup cilantro
- 2 green onions
- ¼ cup olive oil
- 1 tablespoon honey
- 2 cloves garlic
- 1 tsp cumin

DIRECTIONS

1. In a bowl combine all ingredients together and mix well
2. Add dressing and serve

GREEK SALAD

Serves: 2
Prep Time: 5   Minutes
Cook Time: 15   Minutes
Total Time: 20   Minutes

INGREDIENTS

- 1 cup cherry tomatoes
- 1 cucumber
- 1 cup olives
- ¼ red onion
- 1 cup feta
- 1 cup salad dressing

DIRECTIONS

1. In a bowl combine all ingredients together and mix well
2. Add dressing and serve

Serves: **2**
Prep Time: **5**   Minutes
Cook Time: **15**   Minutes
Total Time: **20**   Minutes

INGREDIENTS

- 2 lb. cooked baby potatoes
- 4 slices bacon
- 1 onion
- 1 tablespoon olive oil
- 1 tablespoon mustard
- 1 tsp black pepper

DIRECTIONS

1. In a bowl combine all ingredients together and mix well
2. Add dressing and serve

Serves: *2*
Prep Time: *5*   Minutes
Cook Time: *15* Minutes
Total Time: *20* Minutes

INGREDIENTS

- 1 avocado
- 1 cup tomatoes
- 1 cucumber
- ½ cup cooked corn
- 1 tablespoon cilantro

DIRECTIONS

1. In a bowl combine all ingredients together and mix well
2. Add dressing and serve

Serves: **1**
Prep Time: **5** Minutes
Cook Time: **5** Minutes
Total Time: **10** Minutes

INGREDIENTS

- 1 cup cottage cheese
- 1 cup sour cream
- 2 green onions
- 2 tsp hot sauce
- 1 tsp dill weed
- ¼ tsp garlic powder
- ½ cup blue cheese

DIRECTIONS

1. In a blender add all ingredients together
2. Blend until smooth

3. Serve when ready

GOAT CHEESE DIP

Serves: **1**

Prep Time: **5** Minutes

Cook Time: **5** Minutes

Total Time: **10** Minutes

INGREDIENTS

- 6 oz. goat cheese
- ½ cup ricotta cheese
- 1 scallion
- 1 tsp lemon zest
- 1 tablespoons lemon juice
- 1 tsp black pepper

DIRECTIONS

1. In a blender add all ingredients together
2. Blend until smooth
3. Serve when ready

Serves: **1**
Prep Time: **5**   Minutes
Cook Time: **5**   Minutes
Total Time: **10** Minutes

INGREDIENTS

- ½ cup olive oil
- 2 onions
- 3 shallots
- 1 can sour cream
- 1 tablespoon chives
- 1 tsp salt

DIRECTIONS

1. In a blender add all ingredients together
2. Blend until smooth
3. Serve when ready

Serves: *1*
Prep Time: 5   Minutes
Cook Time: 5   Minutes
Total Time: *10*   Minutes

INGREDIENTS

- 2 avocados
- ½ onion
- ½ cup cilantro
- 1 jalapeno
- ½ cup pepitas
- 2 tablespoons lime juice
- 1 tsp salt

DIRECTIONS

1. In a blender add all ingredients together
2. Blend until smooth

3. Serve when ready

Serves: *1*
Prep Time: 5   Minutes
Cook Time: 5   Minutes
Total Time: *10* Minutes

INGREDIENTS

- 8 oz. cream cheese
- 1 cup Greek yogurt
- ½ cup mayonnaise
- 1 tsp cumin
- 1 tsp paprika
- 1 tsp black pepper
- 1 cup cheddar cheese
- 1 jalapeno pepper

DIRECTIONS

1. **In a blender add all ingredients together**

2. Blend until smooth
3. Serve when ready

SCALLION DIP

Serves: **1**
Prep Time: **5** Minutes
Cook Time: **5** Minutes
Total Time: **10** Minutes

INGREDIENTS

- 1 cup sour cream
- ½ cup mayonnaise
- ¼ cup scallions
- 2 tablespoons dill
- 1 tablespoon lemon zest
- 1 tsp black pepper

DIRECTIONS

1. In a blender add all ingredients together
2. Blend until smooth
3. Serve when ready

PIMENTO CHEESE DIP

Serves: **1**

Prep Time: **5** Minutes

Cook Time: **5** Minutes

Total Time: **10** Minutes

INGREDIENTS

- 1 package cream cheese
- 2 tablespoons lemon juice
- 1 tsp salt
- 1 jar pimientos
- 4 oz. Cheddar cheese
- 4 oz. Jack cheese
- 2 scallions
- 1 tsp black pepper

DIRECTIONS

1. In a blender add all ingredients together

2. Blend until smooth
3. Serve when ready

BLUE-CHEESE DIP

Serves: *1*
Prep Time: *5*   Minutes
Cook Time: *5*   Minutes
Total Time: *10* Minutes

INGREDIENTS

- 1 cup Greek Yogurt
- 1 tablespoon lemon juice
- 1 tsp black pepper
- 1 scallion
- 1 tablespoon parsley
- 3 oz. blue cheese
- 1 cucumber

DIRECTIONS

1. In a blender add all ingredients together
2. Blend until smooth

3. Serve when ready

PIZZA

ZUCCHINI PIZZA

Serves: **6-8**
Prep Time: **10** Minutes

Cook Time: **15** Minutes

Total Time: **25** Minutes

INGREDIENTS

- 1 pizza crust
- ½ cup tomato sauce
- ¼ black pepper
- 1 cup zucchini slices
- 1 cup mozzarella cheese
- 1 cup olives

DIRECTIONS

1. Spread tomato sauce on the pizza crust

2. Place all the toppings on the pizza crust
3. Bake the pizza at 425 F for 12-15 minutes
4. When ready remove pizza from the oven and serve

SALAMI PIZZA

Serves: **6-8**
Prep Time: **10**   Minutes

Cook Time: **15**   Minutes

Total Time: **25**   Minutes

INGREDIENTS

- 1 pizza crust
- ½ cup tomato sauce
- ¼ black pepper
- 1 cup salami slices
- 1 cup Brussel sprouts
- 1 cup mozzarella cheese
- 1 cup olives

DIRECTIONS

1. Spread tomato sauce on the pizza crust
2. Place all the toppings on the pizza crust

3. Bake the pizza at 425 F for 12-15 minutes

4. When ready remove pizza from the oven and serve

Serves: **6-8**
Prep Time: **10**   Minutes
Cook Time: **15**   Minutes
Total Time: **25**   Minutes

INGREDIENTS

- 1 pizza crust
- ½ cup tomato sauce
- ¼ black pepper
- 8-9 prosciutto slices
- 1 cup mozzarella cheese
- 1 cup onion

DIRECTIONS

1. Spread tomato sauce on the pizza crust
2. Place all the toppings on the pizza crust
3. Bake the pizza at 425 F for 12-15 minutes

4. When ready remove pizza from the oven
   and serve

CARROT PIZZA

Serves: **6-8**
Prep Time: **10**   Minutes

Cook Time: **15**   Minutes

Total Time: **25**   Minutes

INGREDIENTS

- 1 pizza crust
- ½ cup tomato sauce
- ¼ black pepper
- 1 cup carrot slices
- 1 cup mozzarella cheese
- 1 cup olives

DIRECTIONS

1. Spread tomato sauce on the pizza crust
2. Place all the toppings on the pizza crust
3. Bake the pizza at 425 F for 12-15 minutes

4. When ready remove pizza from the oven and serve

SQUASH PIZZA

Serves: *6-8*
Prep Time: *10*   Minutes
Cook Time: *15*   Minutes
Total Time: *25*   Minutes

INGREDIENTS

- 1 pizza crust
- ½ cup tomato sauce
- ¼ black pepper
- 1 cup butternut squash
- 1 cup mozzarella cheese
- 1 cup olives

DIRECTIONS

1. Spread tomato sauce on the pizza crust
2. Place all the toppings on the pizza crust
3. Bake the pizza at 425 F for 12-15 minutes

4. When ready remove pizza from the oven and serve

Serves: *6-8*
Prep Time: *10*   Minutes
Cook Time: *15*   Minutes
Total Time: *25*   Minutes

INGREDIENTS

- 1 pizza crust
- ½ cup tomato sauce
- ¼ black pepper
- 3-4 eggs
- 1 cup mozzarella cheese
- 1 cup olives
- 2-3 tomato slices

DIRECTIONS

1. Spread tomato sauce on the pizza crust
2. Place all the toppings on the pizza crust

3. Bake the pizza at 425 F for 12-15 minutes

4. When ready remove pizza from the oven and serve

Serves: **6-8**
Prep Time: **10**   Minutes

Cook Time: **15**   Minutes

Total Time: **25**   Minutes

INGREDIENTS

- 1 pizza crust
- ½ cup tomato sauce
- ¼ black pepper
- 1 cup kale
- 1 cup mozzarella cheese
- 1 cup olives
- 1 cup ricotta

DIRECTIONS

1. Spread tomato sauce on the pizza crust
2. Place all the toppings on the pizza crust

3. Bake the pizza at 425 F for 12-15 minutes
4. When ready remove pizza from the oven and serve

LAMB PIZZA

Serves: *6-8*
Prep Time: *10* Minutes

Cook Time: *15* Minutes

Total Time: *25* Minutes

INGREDIENTS

- 1 pizza crust
- ½ cup tomato sauce
- ¼ black pepper
- 1 cup lamb
- 1 cup mozzarella cheese
- 1 cup olives

DIRECTIONS

1. Spread tomato sauce on the pizza crust
2. Place all the toppings on the pizza crust
3. Bake the pizza at 425 F for 12-15 minutes

4. When ready remove pizza from the oven and serve

Serves: **6-8**
Prep Time: **10**   Minutes
Cook Time: **15**   Minutes
Total Time: **25**   Minutes

INGREDIENTS

- 1 pizza crust
- ½ cup tomato sauce
- ¼ black pepper
- 2 anchovy fillets
- 2 garlic cloves
- 1 cup ricotta
- 2 cups kale
- ¼ cup jalapenos
- 1 cup mozzarella cheese
- 1 cup olives

DIRECTIONS

1. Spread tomato sauce on the pizza crust
2. Place all the toppings on the pizza crust
3. Bake the pizza at 425 F for 12-15 minutes
4. When ready remove pizza from the oven and serve

THANK YOU FOR READING THIS BOOK!

Made in the USA
Monee, IL
01 August 2021